SAILING ON SPIRIT WIND

Midlife Reflections

BY JUDITH PREST

SPIRIT WIND BOOKS

Cindy ~
May your life
be abundant with
love, light & inspiration
as you continue your
journey.

Juditta Frent

SAILING

ON

SPIRIT

WIND

BY JUDITH PREST

This book is dedicated to Grace and John Prest, my parents, who started me on the path.... With thanks to: Miss Sally Longstreth, my high school English teacher, mentor and friend, who continues to teach me about writing; Barbara and Linda, my sisters in spirit; my spouse, Alan and my son Jon; Marilyn Day of WomanWords; Hannelore Hahn and the International Women's Writing Guild and the small army of other wonderful friends and colleagues who have encouraged and supported this project.

Library of Congress 98-96745
ISBN 0-9666891-0-0

©1998
Spirit Wind Books
P.O. Box 15
Duanesburg, NY 12056
e-mail: spwind4@aol.com

Previously published work appearing in this book:
Nightshore, first appeared in "Slightly West",
Winter 1997/1998 Issue

Millennium Musings, first appeared in "Slightly West",
Summer 1998 Issue

Loyalty Oath, first appeared in "Earth's Daughters",
Issue # 51, 1998

Illustrations by Richard B. Carter appear on:
Title Page and Pages 1, 3, 13, 32, 33, 39, 44, 52, and 54.
Photographs by Alan Krieger and Judith Prest
appear on pages 7, 28 and 34.
Book Design by Karen Conway, Conway Creations
www.rpi.edu/~conwam/create.htm
Printed by New Art Printing, Albany, NY 12205

Contents

Introduction

As I began to consider publication of this book—what to put in, what to leave out—I worried about gratuitous sharing, about adding to what I call the "psychological exhibitionism" that abounds at this moment in our culture. My decisions to include some personally revealing pieces were based on what each says about healing and resilience. I believe in the magic of transformation that is available to each of us when we can take the time to reflect on what is good and right with us, when we are able to replace fear with love. I offer this writing in the spirit of passing on wisdom, in the hope that it will spark creativity for others and in gratitude for the gifts that continue to come as I pursue the path of writing and healing.

New Year

a new year
sun's lemon light
flows across blue shadowed snow
in crunching, bone-deep chill
cardinals and sparrows forage
for seed to fuel
their tiny frames
against the cold

a new year
sky washed clean
fresh fields of snow
waiting for tracks
inviting us to continue
the journey

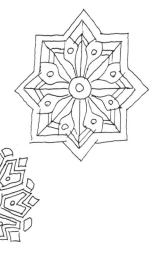

in thin winter light
breath rising like prayer
through clear stillness
light as birdbones
we answer the call
striding into our lives
making tracks
toward the millennium

Spirit Wind

my soul is
reaching
windblown
expanding in rays of violet

barefoot in purple
one foot planted
on cool earth
one foot lifted
to begin the dance
arms flung wide
to catch spirit wind

oh healing light
bring gratitude
bring abundance
bring creativity

let the dance be long
the movement graceful
as circling hawks

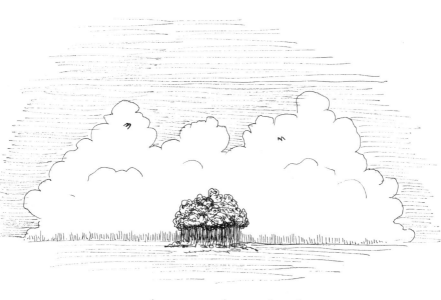

Graceful as circling hawks . . .

Loyalty Oath

under
gathering geese
under sky
frost-scoured blue
I pledge allegiance
to the land
and all the spirits
it holds within

woodthrush and honeysuckle
mushroom and wolf,
frost jewels, ice mandalas
dew-silvered spider web

...to the rustle and hiss
of autumn wind
passing through dry leaves
and pine

...to flapping heron
and plunging hawk
my wild brothers
keepers of the marsh and field

I pledge allegiance to
the First People
earth's keepers
who know land
is not property
living in round time
keeping the long vigil
into dawn

The Calling

through the mist
a loon calls
a clear cry
a calling across
wide waters

a call to reach
into the whirlpool
and pull out what's solid
and sure

a calling
giving voice at last
to the hidden

a calling
to move out of the shadow
the eclipse is finished
sun returns
called back by a wild bird
nesting in my heart

Nightshore

I can see Venus
reflected in tide pools
can feel warm wind
pushing from land to sea

waves gather and crash
slide up the sand
illumined by starlight

in the dark
tides shift, fish feed
shells land among foam and clam bubble
water shapes
and reshapes the sand

we speak of the unspeakable
we poke the underbelly of the night
we seek finally to scour
the dark corners of our lives
with light
bring spirit to dead spaces
give voice to pain and joy
to heal, to liberate
to take flight from this dark shore
moving steadily toward light

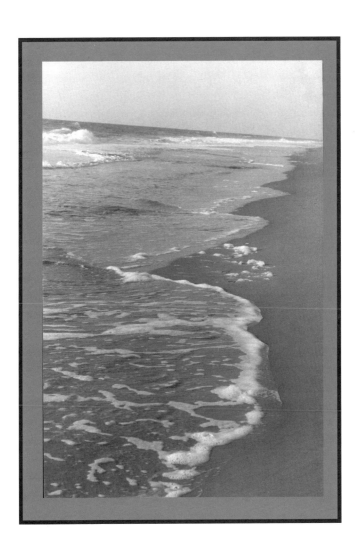

Dry Places

I have been too long
marooned in dry places:
no magic no laughter no tears no soul
hell is not hot
it is cold and dry
filled with bitter dust
fear without comfort, pain without voice
a place of no color
no birdsong no love

dry places are where the critic resides
that ruthless one who rises up
and slices with a keen blade
any shoots of hope
punctures each dream bubble
without giving it a second thought

dry places are inhabited by
the toxic and the sharp
scorpion, rattlesnake
cactus spike, ice shard

marooned in dry places
finally I pray
and God hands me a map

God says
ask and it will come
but not easily
forgiveness and gratitude
mark the trail
you will have to climb alone
but I'll be with you
every step of the way

Anger's House

in anger's house
the walls are thunder
rage ricochets
off the ceiling
the air burns
sears flesh
shrivels spirit

sink to the floor
lay low
crawl beneath
the toxic cloud
out the door

go quickly
fear stunts those
who stay too long
in anger's house
leaves them branded
the scars run deep

cold wind howls
at the window ledge
fire at your back
jump now
save yourself
let anger's house
burn down
without you

The Rape

1.
a 747 crashing
into the sea of my life
leaving a nasty oil slick on top
most of the carnage and damage
lies buried deep
deep below the surface

broken trust
broken dreams
black cold
smothering fear
so far from the light

hide hide
bury it deep
deny deny
make it go away
shame shame
"only you could
bring this on yourself"

2.
slowly
terror retreats
the tide of loathing
recedes into the depths
scar tissue forms
blocking light and life

never the same
never the same
no return, no safe places
ever again

3.
build a shell
body armor
mind fuzz
blot it out
NUMB NUMB

build a false self
on top of the rubble
plant flowers
let it grow over

4.
years pass, life unfolds
finally it seems
there is no moving forward
without a journey
to revisit the disaster scene

decades later
the way is clear
there are markers on the dark waves
beacons only I can see

time to strip down
dive deep into the dark cold
swim through silenced screaming
keep moving through terror
haul out debris
bring it finally
to shore

let in light
let in healing
find the pieces
acknowledge the damage
find peace
move on
FORGIVE LIVE
BELIEVE AGAIN

I Know

I know how sweet maple trees smell when they are in flower and I know how to make helicopters out of maple propellers. I know that the pileated woodpecker sends me a signal so I can look for him in the dead elm tree or on the electric pole on the ridge across the road. I know when to look for that bird.

I know how to search the shallow waters for blue herons and the field edges for wild turkeys as I speed by. This is not the slow and peaceful birdwatching of my parents. In my accelerated life I have learned to look to the side as I fly by, to take in what I can even when I can't stop to savor the view.

I know where trillium blooms, even though I haven't been to see it yet this year. I know how the light spreads at dawn, seeping from below the horizon into the clouds. I know how wind sounds in grass, in pines, through rocks at the tops of mountains. I know how moonlight touches ordinary objects and transforms them.

I know that when I put out sunflower seeds before dawn, cardinals will come to feed at first light, during quiet moments of the day and again at dusk. First the male will come and then the female; sometimes in spring they feed seeds to each other. I know that if I keep putting food out, the rose breasted grosbeak will come later this season. I know that when I pay attention to the earth I am rewarded with peace and well being. I know that time will pass, sometimes stretching like sticky taffy between my fingers, sometimes in storm-driven gusts. I know that healing occurs for all hurts if we are able to stand back from the wound and allow the spirit to do its work. I know that our souls need food more than our bodies and that mine needs regular meals of quiet, nature, reflection and prayer.

Prayer as I practice it is very different from the ceremonial forms of church and synagogue. Those have their own power and their own place. My prayer is more of the sweaty, white knuckled variety: "Please God, I'm pinned against the wall again by fear. Please help me find and hold the lines of love to pull myself free". I know these prayers are answered always. I know because just the act of praying gives me the strength to pull the plug on that awful current of terror that pins me down. Because of this, I know that walls and limitations are often illusions. I am beginning to understand what they meant when they said faith can move mountains.

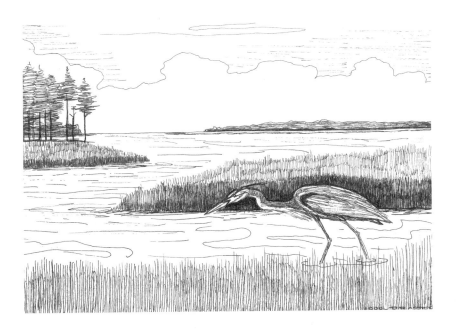

Resilience

sometimes a makeshift tabernacle
decorated with porcelain bowls
and mosaic floors
is all that stands
between me and devastation

sometimes only a single
magnolia blossom
anchors me to terra firma

sometimes my muse
plays peek-a-boo with me
in the inner sanctum
until we both collapse
in giggle frenzy
laughter lifting me high
above the reach of earthquakes
and rogue waves

by these fragile links
strength builds
words flow
food for the journey
wine for the soul

Labyrinth

one foot follows the other
along this thin serpentine path
I am aware of other trails
just next to the one I walk

we walk alone
and together
in full silence
under soft evening light
wind hissing in pines

bare feet move through sandy grass
feeling that root energy reaching
down to water
up to light
passing through the soles of my feet
to the core of my being

curves and switchbacks
each step tracing the pattern
turning turning
round like life

it is hard to balance
on this narrow path
yet I keep moving ahead
now to center, now outward
one step at a time
bathed in gold light
an inner compass
leading me home

Time

Give me
dream time
time out-of-mind

Oh Time, you
ghost dancer, windwalker
shape shifter
trickster:
Bring me your gifts
tell me your secrets
Let me flow in and out
with the tides

Dance with me
while the nights are short
Fly with me
when the days are long
and full of light

Teach me
to live in round-time
Sun over the mountain time
Make me wise
let my days be unnumbered
my hours uncounted
Help me remember the secret:
Time is
no big deal
to the soul

Millennium Musings

I am obsessed with
time passing
generations
rings in trees
all of us growing older
layers of experience exposed
like earth layers in a canyon

I imagine
limp watches
calendars turned to Jell-O
as we swim, trudge
slither and dance
through time

is time round?
does it bear down
on us like
a glacier
or an avalanche?

or does it spiral
softly down
through the ages
rocks to sand
flesh to bone
pushing up green spears
through frosty earth
again and again
while God applauds?

I Remember

I remember colors on sand, reflected from the sky that appear when a wave recedes. I remember first noticing this on a December day in college when Linda and I drove to Stone Harbor. It was a Sunday and it was cold and sunny. I remember how the tree shadows lay across the road creating dizzy-making visual effects as we drove. I remember hard yellow light slanting through bare trees, hitting the blacktop as we puttered across the New Jersey flats, two kids playing hooky from life; two young women with so much life ahead and so much history to come to terms with.

I remember Stone Harbor; the Stone Harbor of my childhood, that smelled of salt marsh - that sharp stink of marsh mud and sea life at low tide. It was a sea town with empty blocks still, sandy lots where bay bushes and scrub pines grew, egrets roosting in some. I remember osprey nests on top of dead trees poking up from the marsh. The birds were always the center of these short coastal journeys with my parents; at Stone Harbor we had about equal amounts of beach time and bird time.

I remember the overnight trip I took there with my mother when I was eighteen. That summer I felt washed up and I suppose I literally was - washed up on the shore of young adulthood after the violent storm of my adolescence. Grace and I stayed at a rooming house. We got up early and walked the beach together. I remember that particular Stone Harbor visit as a time when my mother and I were sort of equals, when we had moments of adult-like companionship and sharing for the first time.

I remember that when I was eighteen my mother really tried to reach out to me. On that trip to Stone Harbor we connected. At other times, I felt bewildered and responded blankly to her efforts. Now I think I was wondering where she was when I was floundering and lost, that some part of me thought, "NOW you want to pay attention???". In the present as this thought unfolds, I still feel the sting, but I also know that I have yet to parent a teenager.

That time we were there to visit Grace's friend Ethel whose elderly father owned a house in Stone Harbor and whose sister always came from California to meet her there. I remember being on the beach with Ethel's niece, Valerie. She was eighteen like me and we remembered each other from other times when our parents had all been at the beach. She was golden and innocent. A ripe peach of a California girl, she seemed to be untouched. The contrast between us was striking and I was put off by her sunny attitude, her open approach to life. When I considered myself next to her, I felt very old. Staggering under the weight of recent traumas, I felt battered then but didn't know it. At the time I just felt sour and worn out.

I felt much younger that bare treed day in college when Linda and I abandoned our studying and headed for the beach in her black VW bug. As I write this so many years later I feel younger yet, maybe refreshed and healed is more accurate. I am learning how to get out of my own way and allow life to unfold. I am learning to trust the universe and my own wisdom. I know now that I can ask for help and it will come—not always in the form I expect, but it will be there. I can count on it, as surely as one wave follows the next, each one leaving sky colors along the shoreline as it recedes.

Motherhood Trilogy # 1
To My First One

little spark of life
phantom child long gone
I light a candle for you now

I hold the pain
of your brief existence
deep in my body
cushioned against sharp edges
safe from cold wind

little spirit
long moved on
the dues of your going
paid in the currency
of tears and blood
scalpels, gauze
and infertility

phantom child
there is no measure
for this loss
no accounting
can be made for
the time it took
for me to see you
standing in shadow
at the borders of my life

waiting for welcome
waiting for forgiveness
waiting to take your place in my heart

Motherhood Trilogy # 2
For Gloria

sometimes I feel my arms extended
through time and space
reaching for
your outstretched hands

no doubt what has brought me joy
has brought you sorrow
through your hard choices
I became a mother

two lives divided
by gulf and border
by miles of dry country
connected by sorrow and joy

I dream our hands clasped
tan and brown
bridging canyons of pain
the raw power of our loss and love
generating strong white light
to protect our son
and illuminate his path

when I look into his eyes
when he smiles
when I greet him in the morning
you are there
a faint shape
at the edge of my vision
reminding me
that letting go
is an act of love

Motherhood Trilogy # 3
For Jon

you stand midpoint in childhood
and I remember
your baby cheeks
our songs and stories
your toddler delight
in pine cones and fireflies

I see myself
weeping in the road
tears falling on the yellow line
the kindergarten bus disappearing
around the bend
removing you from
my circle of protection in a new way
transporting you into your own world

now you navigate the larger waters
of third grade
and I remember how you felt
in my arms that first time
lighter than the cat

I remember holding you those first weeks
the wait finally over
chanting "Sweet One,
you're the one
I waited for".
willing you to
soak up love and welcome
through all the pores of your being

I remember joy at your first steps
then being stricken with the knowledge
that all steps after these would be
steps away from me
into your own life
if I do the job right

I see you now
with wonder and gratitude:
your gentleness with animals
your concentration
as you draw a picture
your moments of total glee

I wonder and worry
how you will negotiate
the territory ahead
those years from 12 to 20
that nearly broke me
on their rocks

I pray that my love will be a beacon
that my fear will not
obstruct your path
that you will emerge strong and sure
capable and connected
a man of substance

Memory's Wind

as the road spins
under my tires
memory's wind stirs
hisses
roars
stretching time
reshaping my heartspace

under the force of this wind
seasons spin
the dead live again
words unuttered
can now be spoken

memory's wind blows
scraps of past lives
through
my now

a relentless sirocco
sweeping from hotter regions
swells
presses
splits open the present
flattens all structures
exposing the bones of truth
revealing what will stand
when the wind falls

Turning Points

all mine are vital
bound up in blood
in tears
opening to receive
or to relinquish
struggle always
an essential element

wind wrestling
wave dodging
too much duck and cover
except when
not enough

turning points evoke
memories of clenched fingers
squeezing meaning out
grasping for essence
sometimes crushing the petals
in the effort
to preserve the scent

On Becoming A "Grown-up"
for my father

your hands in the hospital
thin now but still huge
one holding mine
through those last nights
anchoring your spirit
in the pause before flight

cold stale air, fluorescent light
through the relentless hum
of the night hospital
your voice faintly tracing
the map of your life
one more time

I see myself then: your daughter
a grown woman
not yet a mother
no longer a girl,
walking with you to the edge
blinded by tears and fear
receiving my first lessons
in the immortality of love
as you helped me cross
the last boundary of childhood

Death Watch

hospital nights
the walls breathe
life's machinery
beeps and blinks
even as death waits
in the corner of the room

watching for that moment
when the spirit will rise
and it will
even as we reach our living hands
across the abyss
even as we seek to
follow with our hearts

breath has left with spirit
only your form remains
leaving us forever changed
by our journey with you
to the gate

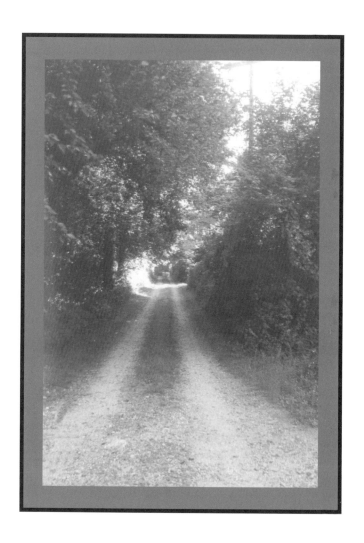

389 County Road

The road that leads off the main road to the house in Bear is now paved. Until I was sixteen it was a dirt road. I know that our lane came three-tenths of a mile and six telephone poles in from the main road because that is how my mother always gave people directions to our house.

At first I was driven and later walked down that road twice a day, to and from the school bus stop. In the spring the road was often muddy. By late summer it would be bumpy, washboarded with ruts that made the car stutter along and rattled our teeth. There was a large and beautiful tulip poplar just across from where our lane came out. I remember it lying ripped out on its side, still budding, in my sixteenth spring when they were tearing out trees to widen and pave the road.

Halfway between our lane and the main road was an abandoned cemetery that belonged to a church several miles away. The graveyard was a place of mystery and intrigue; a place to hurry past on dark days and a place to explore with brave friends on Saturday mornings. The lane crosses railroad tracks. Sometimes trains would stop at the highway and block our lane. Several times I had to climb across train car couplings to get out to the road in time for the school bus.

The lane was dirt and gravel and would get rutted and nearly impassable from time to time. Loads of gravel were brought in to even it out. Before the gravel there were more interesting stones in the lane. I remember earlier walks at age three, four and five with my mother, picking up stones.

29

She taught me that the ones with rings all the way around them were lucky stones—we made wishes on them.

I remember the first time I drove the 1960 two-toned blue Rambler station wagon down the lane, my father at my side. I was quite taken with the serious responsibility of driving and was concentrating hard on shifting into second gear with the three speed on-the-column transmission. My father suddenly yelled, "Left, Left!!". Since I still have trouble with right and left, I froze when he did this and looked up in time to see a cherry tree coming at us in slow motion.

We pushed the tree over and put a large dent in the bumper. My father, ever game, was ready to go on, but I was finished for the day. However, it wasn't long until I was taking the lane at forty miles an hour, trying unsuccessfully to knock off a chicken or two on my way up the hill.

Three times in my memory snow closed the road. The first was during the winter of first grade. A big blizzard cut off power for three days. No plows came so my father and the Gicker boys dug us out using peach baskets for shovels, not only the lane but also the dirt road, all the way to the main road.

During Christmas vacation when I was fourteen, a large snow came. The road was not plowed out for several days. Our guests for Christmas dinner had to park at the tavern on the main road and walk in on the railroad tracks. That season I remember walking the unplowed road by moonlight to visit my friend Barbie who lived two fields away. The fields were too snowy for trudging that night.

The third "snowing in" came in February of 1983, the night after my father died. By morning, all the roads in the state were closed and we knew we weren't getting out any time soon, even for a funeral. It felt satisfying that my dad's passage was marked by a large natural event. It felt right that everything had to grind to a halt for a few days. My father's death marked the beginning of my "long good bye" to the land which continues at this writing.

The view from the bottom of the lane is sky framed by trees. The house is not visible at that point, creating a sense of heading into unmapped territory as one starts to drive up the lane. On the rare occasions when I fly in, there are always laborious explanations at the airport shuttle desk that no, there is not a development nearby, we'll have to rely on route numbers and road names to get there. When we finally turn into the lane, I wonder what the driver is thinking as we head through the trees into the great unknown.

Now after living in other places for many years, whenever I drive up the lane, I am struck with gratitude for having grown up in such a unique and magical setting. I am also grateful that my son has spent enough time here to have clear memories of the road, the railroad tracks and the lane leading to Grandma's house.

For Grace On Her 80th
A Snapshot From Your Daughter....

Grace has been a practicing eccentric all her life. Many people think the poem "When I Am Old I Shall Wear Purple" was written with her in mind.

Grace taught me to love nature, stand up for what I believe in and to see the humor in things. She excels at networking. She has an incredible sense of the ridiculous and is very good at skewering the pompous. She loves birds and words and silver, studied plants and bugs.

I remember when the house was filled with cigar boxes containing insects impaled on long pins. She taught me to observe and appreciate small wonders. Grace has a sense of the universal and has often said she's content knowing she's a tiny speck in the great scheme of stars, planets, nature and life.

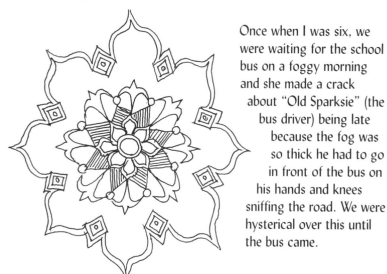

Once when I was six, we were waiting for the school bus on a foggy morning and she made a crack about "Old Sparksie" (the bus driver) being late because the fog was so thick he had to go in front of the bus on his hands and knees sniffing the road. We were hysterical over this until the bus came.

Grace appreciates bathroom humor and great writing. I often thought if she'd been raised in different times she would have been a journalist. She writes well, thinks quickly, can get anybody talking about anything and has a healthy skepticism for "bureaucrat-speak".

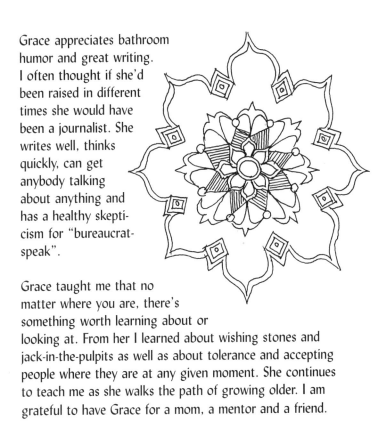

Grace taught me that no matter where you are, there's something worth learning about or looking at. From her I learned about wishing stones and jack-in-the-pulpits as well as about tolerance and accepting people where they are at any given moment. She continues to teach me as she walks the path of growing older. I am grateful to have Grace for a mom, a mentor and a friend.

Message To My Son

once I was young
everything was new
and I was bold and terrified
as I swam far out
in the sea of my life

beyond the breakers
beyond the jetty
into the realm of
riptides and sharks

and because I believed
love couldn't follow
I was alone in deep water
nearly drowned

you will never be
beyond the reach
of my love

sometimes it will seem so
sometimes you will wish it
sometimes you will find yourself
in places I can't go
even in my imagination

but even there
my love will follow
as long as you
believe it will

Winter Solstice

I long for the light
flowing from higher places
water to a parched soul

as December darkens
spirals into
winter night
sun enters and exits with exquisite color
dawning late, dimming early
leaving only cold starlight

in bone cracking cold
we stoke our souls' fires
with prayer, with hope
with evergreen and candle flame

soon comes solstice
to begin the turning
of the sun's tide
from dark to bright

Totem

raven wing
black pearl
iridescent
glow blue
shiny sharp air-knife
moonwind's raucous brother
sassy wisdom
sharp eyed brilliance

beaked phantom
messenger of spirit
you know me
you seek the hidden
and the shiny

together we will
uncover more

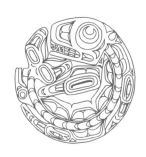

Prayer of the Alligator

oh these long hot afternoons
of wet blanket air
muddy bank and murky
swirling water

send me something I can get my teeth into
let me feel that satisfying crunch
as my jaws clamp down on dinner

send me a fat creature
it doesn't have to be too slow
just let it wander
into the path of my golden vision
and I will do the rest

in the heat I wait
for an answer to this prayer
while I wait I'll meditate on
fly buzz and algae
listening to swamp moss tendrils
entwining with earth and treebark

as I wait I'll imagine
the spirit of my supper
and give thanks to the creature
who will nourish me

April

spring swoops in
from the south
heralded by robin and crocus

under gentle rain
earth smells deep
like roots

last year's leaves
still crackle
on the forest floor
as new life
pushes above the frost line

woodcocks buzz and twitter
in the evening fields
redwings grace the swamps again
the owl hunts at dawn

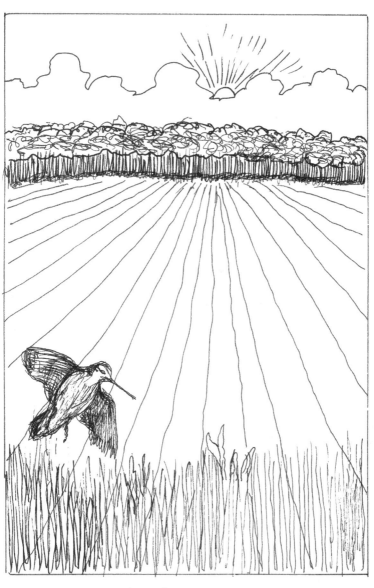

Woodcocks buzz and twitter
in the evening fields . . .

Thundergust

in the place where wind gathers
dark clouds swirl and mumble
releasing sharp gusts
that rip tender leaves from branches
hurling them down
limp and spent along the blacktop

in the space of several heartbeats
bright day is obscured
the lake goes black
turns a blind eye skyward

wind hisses and shrieks
breaking trees
sky meets earth
threat becomes a kept promise
as rain and lightning
fill the air

nothing left but
surrender
to wind and water
pray hard for deliverance
through the flash and rumble

caught on a back road
sheets of rain
falling trees
clouds crossing the pavement
just ahead
I keep driving
a moving target
the car suddenly a fragile vessel

this day trip deepens
into yet another lesson
about fear
and faith

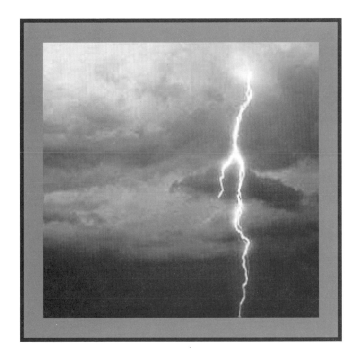

Pond At Dawn

pale sky
sunrise and moonset
balanced
across dawn

clouds flame
mist rises and drifts
under the surface frogs wait
bass turn
flashing silver sides

dragonfly skims the surface
rattles and clicks
while heron
stalks the edge
seeking slow frogs

cardinal's call reaches
through trees
across drifts of Queen Anne's Lace
a rich whistle
full of scarlet promise

Poet In The Jury Box

you will
consider the evidence
they said
and only the evidence
presented by witnesses
in this courtroom

you will not consider
all the lives undone
by this breaking of the law

you will not consider
the sound of gunfire
the silence of death
or the trajectory of bullets
mapping fracture lines
across so many lives

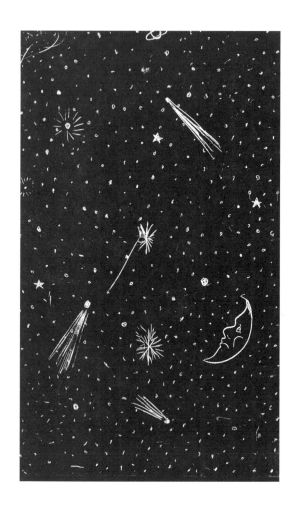

Stars

pinpricks of light
crossing the night sky
wheeling, turning
sparks hurled forth
God's breath
condensing
in deep space

the elements in us
came from the stars
the sea beats in our blood
we are mirrors for the universe
dancing with God
our lives like little comets
making light trails
between the stars

Moon Prayer

tide puller, light bearer
you count the rhythm
for our brief dance
beneath the stars

moonfire: burning like dry ice
what revolutionary acts
have been sparked
by your silver flame?

crones rejoice
when your face shines full
round as the sacred cycles
of water and blood
your light the color
of spider webs
weaving souls together
a bond stronger
than tempered steel

once men landed
with machines and flags
their heavy boots
marking your surface
in the name of
"discovery"

still your face remains
unchanged
shining for us
sending silvered sunlight
tempering
our dark nights
calling the beat
as we dance on

Light

My relationship with light is complex and vital. First there is
physical light, the light from the sun and from the stars
reaching us daily from distance so far it is measured in light
years. Starlight so ancient that its source has flamed out
long before human sight records its presence.

Those tides of light called seasons are directly linked with
my vital energy; it runs low and concentrated in the dark
of winter, expands as light returns with spring. My spirit
needs light like my body needs air: Flat light on snow in a
Wyoming blizzard, all depth erased, sky and earth and air
becoming one seamless fabric of white, accented only by
fence posts and telephone poles. The amber light of a long
summer sunset that catches and holds my heart inside its
center. Green sunlight filtered through new leaves, plants
glowing emerald as sunlight fuels the process of photosyn-
thesis. Blue shadows on snowdrifts, the subzero sparks
ignited by sun hitting freshly fallen snow. The red shapes
behind my eyelids on the noon beach in August.

Then there is moonlight, that silver fire, interrupting sleep,
inviting the wildwoman to come out and dance. Moon light
calls forth the crone in me, her outlines growing stronger
with every repetition. Moonlight makes the dark safe, helps
us uncover magic in the ordinary.

Then there is the light we can see only with our hearts
and spirits: the glow of love, kindness, forgiveness and
gratitude. This is the light that leads us through our human
lives, the inner light that we all carry, that was meant to be
shared. This light grows within us as we reach out to God,
and all manifestations of God—the natural world, all beings

47

in it, our own higher selves. I believe our world (and maybe the universe) operates on the polarities of love and fear.

Each time one of us is able to choose love over fear, our inner light grows brighter, our souls expand and become closer to God. These are the cords of light that Carlos Casteneda saw in his Don Juan adventures, this is the light that the Bible warns not to hide under a bushel, the light Nelson Mandela was talking about in his inaugural address, "it is our light not our darkness that most frightens us". Wise people from many cultures understand the properties of light and dark.

I believe these universal principles transcend religious and ethnic lines, are true across the ages and will ultimately save us or at least lead us to find our truest, highest selves. This is how I understand spiritual growth. I don't believe we can teach it or that we should preach about it—it is one of those things we learn by example and experience.

So much of my life up to this point has been a search for what feels right and true for me; a struggle to stop doing things that impede spiritual growth, to learn how to project my energy lovingly instead of holding it clenched up in a futile effort to hold back fear. Everything in my life has led me to where I am now and I am grateful for all of it. I hope my struggles have given me wisdom to handle ongoing challenges with more grace and patience, with more faith. I want to proceed through the second half of my life in love and in light, one step at a time.

After The Conference

I have come home to my true country
I know the language
the culture is my own

I have come home to join
the company of women:
women who write, women who dream
standing up at last
to be who we are

so many survivors
of private holocausts:
rape, battering,
discrimination,
devastating despair

some of us have left
ashes still smoldering
to be here
present in our own lives
bearing witness

we are phoenix
we are eagles
here in the company of women
we explore our hearts
mapping
the geography of spirit

here we take wing
we dream
we write and heal
name our Muse
thank our Goddess
and reclaim our souls

Legacy

remember me when the tide turns
in rain, in sun, in ice patterns
in the dragonfly skimming over pondwater

remember how fiercely I loved
my family and my friends

remember loyalty and kindness
remember me for being funny
and feisty and strong and brave

let the legacy be one of caring
bridging gaps, seeking
to create understanding
across wide chasms

remember me as someone
who lived large
tried to be honest
faced her flaws and fears

remember me
as one who dreamed of healing
for herself, humanity, the planet
willing a legacy of love and hope

The Geography of Loss

Waking with dust in my mouth
pain in my heart
I come slowly to consciousness

the reality of loss
develops slowly:
a Polaroid of devastation
locking grief in for the day
as first the edges
then the center of the picture
come clear

vacant houses
place settings before empty chairs
formless piles of folded clothes
silence reverberates

desolate peaks rise
in murky distance
endless desert
sandstone arroyos
earth's bones exposed
by bitter wind

this land
is full of dust

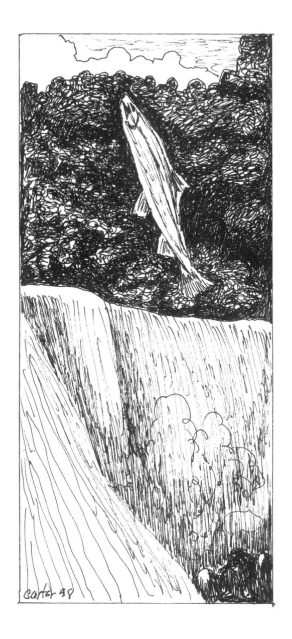

Magic and Prayer

I send a prayer
for the faithful green
returning
after winter has held all
in its harsh embrace

and to migrating birds
returning north
their long flight
a prayer of wings
holding the wind
lifting lifting
finding home

magic and prayer
are linked
one calls forth the other
in a spiral dance
to the beat of waves
the rhythm of seasons

it is magic
that propels the salmon
slicing through miles of blank ocean
to hone in on the exact inlet
returning to its birthriver
to spawn and die
completing the cycle
in familiar waters

like our human souls
this sacred circle
holding god's voice and
a prayer to earth

Sailing on Spirit Wind

today my name is firewalker
traveling into fear's heart
with a blowtorch
I reclaim my power

yesterday my name was
nightmare hurricane
and I thundered across oceans
flattening everything in my path

today I journey
deep into the dark
and back again
retracing the path
retelling the story
making sure it ends well
this time

someday I will call myself raven
sailing on spirit wind
and nothing will ever
hold me down again

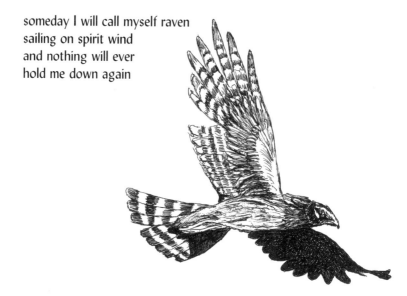

About the author:

Judith Prest wrote poetry through high school and college, then took a 25 year detour through graduate school, career, marriage and parenthood, returning to writing in 1996. She has been a member of the International Women's Writing Guild (IWWG) since 1996, and a member of WomanWords, the Capital District IWWG cluster since it began in early 1997.

Ms. Prest was born and raised in Delaware. She is a graduate of The Evergreen State College, Olympia, Washington and SUNY Albany's School of Social Welfare. Her experiences as a child care worker, taxi driver, world traveler, teacher/counselor and parent have expanded her education, which continues....

She currently works as a Prevention Coordinator in Schenectady County schools, providing training to students, faculty and staff. Judith Prest lives in rural upstate New York with her husband Alan Krieger, their son, Jon and various furry family members of the canine and feline persuasion.